WHAT YOUR BABY NEEDS

Understanding and Communicating Meaning to Unspoken Reactions of Infants for New Moms and Dads

Olivia Jones

Table of Contents

Introduction

Understanding Your Baby's Needs

Parenting is a journey unlike any other, filled with joy, challenges, and a myriad of emotions. At the heart of this journey lies a profound responsibility: understanding and meeting the needs of your baby. From the moment they enter the world, babies communicate their needs through cries, gestures, and subtle cues. As parents, it is our role to decipher these signals and provide the love, care, and support our little ones require to thrive.

Winter's Story:

Winter was a first-time mother filled with excitement and anticipation as she welcomed her baby boy into the world. Like many new parents, she was eager to provide her son with everything he needed to grow and flourish. However, amidst the sleepless nights and endless diaper changes, Winter found herself struggling to understand her baby's needs.

In those early days, her son's cries seemed like a mysterious code she couldn't decipher. Was he hungry, tired, or uncomfortable? Despite her best efforts, Winter often felt overwhelmed and unsure of how to soothe her crying baby.

Determined to forge a deeper connection with her son, Winter embarked on a journey of discovery. She spent countless hours reading books, seeking advice from other parents, and observing her baby's behavior with keen attention. Slowly but surely, Winter began to unravel the mystery of her son's needs.

Through trial and error, Winter learned to recognize the subtle cues that indicated her baby's hunger, fatigue, and discomfort. She discovered that a gentle touch, a soothing lullaby, or a warm embrace could work wonders in calming her baby's cries and bringing him comfort.

As Winter's understanding grew, so did her bond with her son. She found herself tuning into his needs with an intuition that seemed to come naturally. Whether it was a need for cuddles, a change of scenery, or simply a moment of quiet reassurance, Winter was there, ready to respond with love and care.

With each passing day, Winter marveled at the unique individual her son was becoming. She embraced the challenges of parenthood with a newfound confidence, knowing that she had the power to nurture and support her baby through every stage of development.

Winter's story is a testament to the transformative power of understanding your baby's needs. By taking the time to listen, observe, and respond with sensitivity, parents can forge a deep and meaningful connection with their little ones. In the pages that follow, we will explore the essential elements of meeting your baby's needs, offering guidance, insights, and practical strategies to help you navigate the joys and challenges of parenthood. Together, let us embark on this journey of discovery, as we unlock the secrets of what your baby truly needs.

Chapter 1

Physical Well-being

From the moment your baby is born, their physical well-being becomes a top priority. Providing them with the foundation for healthy growth and development requires attention to various aspects of their care, including nutrition, sleep, and safety. In this chapter, we will delve into each of these areas, exploring the importance of proper nutrition, sleep essentials for infants, and creating a safe environment for your little one to thrive.

Nutrition: A Foundation for Growth

Nutrition plays a vital role in supporting your baby's overall health and development. During the first year of life, babies experience rapid growth and development, making it crucial to provide them with the essential nutrients they need to thrive. Whether you choose to breastfeed or formula-feed your baby, ensuring they receive adequate nutrition is paramount.

Breastfeeding is often hailed as the gold standard for infant nutrition, offering a unique blend of antibodies, vitamins, and nutrients that support your baby's immune system and overall health. The World Health Organization recommends exclusive breastfeeding for the first six months of life, followed by the introduction of complementary foods alongside continued breastfeeding for up to two years or beyond.

For mothers who are unable to breastfeed or choose not to do so, formula feeding provides a nutritious alternative. Formulas are designed to mimic the composition of breast milk, providing babies with the essential nutrients they need to thrive. It is important to follow the manufacturer's instructions when preparing and feeding formula to ensure your baby receives the appropriate amount and consistency.

As your baby grows and transitions to solid foods, it is essential to introduce a variety of nutrient-rich foods to support their continued growth and development. Aim to offer a balanced diet that includes fruits, vegetables, whole grains, lean proteins, and healthy fats. Introducing a diverse range of foods early on can help cultivate healthy eating habits and preferences that will last a lifetime.

In addition to providing nutritious foods, it is important to pay attention to your baby's feeding cues and respond accordingly. Babies have tiny stomachs and may need to feed frequently, especially in the early weeks and months of life. Look for signs of hunger such as rooting, sucking on fists, or making smacking noises, and offer feedings as needed.

As your baby grows and becomes more active, they may begin to show interest in self-feeding and exploring different textures and flavors. Encourage their curiosity and independence by offering age-appropriate finger foods and allowing them to explore and experiment with feeding themselves.

Remember that every baby is unique, and their nutritional needs may vary. Consult with your pediatrician or a registered dietitian if you have any concerns or questions about your baby's feeding habits or nutritional requirements. By providing your baby with a foundation of healthy nutrition from the start, you are setting them up for a lifetime of good health and well-being.

Sleep Essentials for Infants

Sleep is essential for your baby's growth, development, and overall well-being. During the first few months of life, newborns typically sleep for short periods throughout the day and night, waking frequently for feedings and comfort. As your baby grows, their sleep patterns will evolve, eventually consolidating into more predictable naps and longer stretches of nighttime sleep.

Establishing healthy sleep habits from the start can help your baby develop good sleep hygiene and promote better sleep for the entire family. While every baby is different, there are some general guidelines and strategies you can use to support healthy sleep habits:

Create a consistent bedtime routine: Establishing a soothing bedtime routine can help signal to your baby that it is time to wind down and prepare for sleep. This may include activities such as a warm bath, gentle massage, reading a bedtime story, or singing a lullaby.

Encourage daytime naps: Naps are essential for your baby's growth and development, providing them with the restorative rest they need to recharge. Aim for age-appropriate nap schedules and create a quiet, dark, and comfortable sleep environment to promote restful naps throughout the day.

Practice safe sleep practices: The American Academy of Pediatrics recommends placing babies on their backs to sleep to reduce the risk of sudden infant death syndrome (SIDS). Ensure your baby's sleep environment is free from hazards such as loose bedding, pillows, and soft toys, and use a firm mattress with a fitted sheet.

Respond to your baby's cues: Pay attention to your baby's sleep cues and respond promptly when they show signs of tiredness. Look for yawning, rubbing their eyes, or becoming fussy, and offer them the opportunity to rest in a quiet and soothing environment.

Be patient and consistent: Developing healthy sleep habits takes time and patience. Be consistent in your approach to sleep and provide gentle reassurance and comfort to your baby as they learn to self-soothe and settle themselves to sleep.

It is important to remember that babies' sleep patterns can vary widely and may change frequently, especially during periods of growth, teething, or developmental milestones. Be flexible and responsive to your baby's changing needs, and seek support from healthcare professionals or sleep consultants if you encounter persistent sleep challenges.

By prioritizing healthy sleep habits and creating a supportive sleep environment for your baby, you can help them get the restorative rest they need to thrive and grow.

Ensuring a Safe Environment

Creating a safe environment for your baby is paramount to their well-being and development. From the moment they come into the world, babies are curious explorers, eager to learn about their surroundings through touch, sight, and sound. As parents, it is our responsibility to safeguard them from potential hazards and create a secure space where they can grow and thrive.

Here are some essential tips for ensuring a safe environment for your baby:

Babyproof your home: Take proactive steps to babyproof your home by securing furniture, covering electrical outlets, and installing safety gates at the top and bottom of stairs. Keep small objects, choking hazards, and toxic substances out of reach, and anchor heavy furniture and appliances to prevent tipping.

Supervise closely: Never leave your baby unattended, especially in situations where they could be at risk of injury. Keep a close eye on them during playtime, bath time, and mealtime, and provide constant supervision when they are in unfamiliar environments or around pets.

Practice safe sleep: Follow the American Academy of Pediatrics' guidelines for safe sleep practices, including placing your baby on their back to sleep, using a firm mattress with a fitted sheet, and keeping their sleep environment free from hazards such as loose bedding and soft toys.

Use age-appropriate gear: Choose age-appropriate gear and equipment for your baby, including car seats, strollers, high chairs, and baby carriers. Make sure these items are properly installed and used according to the manufacturer's instructions to ensure your baby's safety.

Educate yourself: Stay informed about common childhood injuries and accidents, and learn how to respond in emergency situations. Take a pediatric first aid and CPR course, and keep essential supplies such as a thermometer, bandages, and saline solution on hand in case of minor injuries or illnesses.

Childproof your yard: If you have outdoor space, take steps to childproof your yard by installing fences, locking gates, and removing potential hazards such as sharp objects, toxic plants, and pools or bodies of water.

Stay vigilant: As your baby grows and becomes more mobile, reassess your home environment regularly to identify and address any new safety risks. Be proactive in addressing potential hazards and take steps to prevent accidents before they occur.

Creating a safe environment for your baby requires diligence, foresight, and ongoing attention to detail. By taking proactive steps to safeguard your home and educate yourself about potential risks, you can create a secure space where your baby can explore, learn, and thrive safely.

Chapter 2

Emotional Development

Emotional development is a cornerstone of your baby's overall well-being, laying the groundwork for healthy relationships, resilience, and self-regulation throughout their lives. In this chapter, we will explore the critical components of emotional development, including building a secure attachment, recognizing and responding to emotional cues, and encouraging positive social interactions.

Building a Secure Attachment

Attachment refers to the deep emotional bond that forms between a baby and their primary caregiver, typically beginning in infancy. A secure attachment provides the foundation for healthy social and emotional development, fostering feelings of safety, trust, and security in the child.

There are several key principles to keep in mind when building a secure attachment with your baby:

Responsiveness: Respond promptly and consistently to your baby's needs, whether they are crying for comfort, seeking reassurance, or expressing joy. By being attuned to your baby's cues and providing sensitive and nurturing responses, you can help them feel secure and valued.

Physical closeness: Physical touch is a powerful way to communicate love and affection to your baby. Engage in frequent skin-to-skin contact, cuddling, and gentle rocking to promote feelings of warmth and security.

Eye contact and communication: Make eye contact with your baby during interactions, and respond to their coos, babbles, and facial expressions with enthusiasm and warmth. This back-and-forth exchange helps your baby feel seen and understood, strengthening the bond between you.

Predictability and routine: Establishing predictable routines and rituals can provide a sense of stability and security for your baby. Consistent bedtime routines, mealtimes, and daily rituals help your baby feel safe and confident in their environment.

Emotional regulation: Model healthy emotional regulation by expressing your own feelings in a calm and constructive manner. When your baby sees you managing stress, frustration, and other emotions effectively, they learn valuable coping skills that they can apply in their own lives.

By prioritizing responsiveness, physical closeness, communication, predictability, and emotional regulation, you can lay the foundation for a secure attachment with your baby, fostering a deep and lasting bond that promotes their emotional well-being.

Recognizing and Responding to Emotional Cues

Babies communicate their emotions through a variety of cues, ranging from facial expressions and body language to vocalizations and gestures. As a parent, it is important to tune into these cues and respond sensitively to your baby's emotional needs.

Some common emotional cues to watch for include:

Smiling: A genuine smile indicates happiness and contentment, signaling that your baby feels safe and secure in their environment.

Crying: Crying is your baby's primary means of communication, signaling a variety of needs such as hunger, discomfort, fatigue, or overstimulation. Respond promptly to your baby's cries and try to identify and address the underlying cause.

Frowning or furrowing brows: These facial expressions may indicate discomfort, frustration, or sadness. Offer comfort and reassurance to help your baby feel safe and supported.

Coos and babbling: Vocalizations such as cooing and babbling are your baby's way of expressing joy and engagement. Respond with enthusiastic attention and engage in reciprocal vocalizations to encourage communication and bonding.

By paying close attention to your baby's emotional cues and responding with empathy and sensitivity, you can foster a sense of security and trust, laying the groundwork for healthy emotional development.

Encouraging Positive Social Interactions

Social interactions play a crucial role in your baby's emotional development, helping them learn to navigate relationships, understand social cues, and develop empathy and compassion for others. As your baby grows and begins to interact more with the world around them, there are several ways you can encourage positive social interactions:

Facilitate peer interactions: Arrange playdates with other babies and toddlers to provide opportunities for socialization and peer interaction. Encourage cooperative play and sharing, and model positive social behaviors such as taking turns and expressing gratitude.

Engage in joint activities: Participate in interactive activities such as reading books, singing songs, and playing games with your baby. These shared experiences foster bonding and communication, helping your baby feel connected and valued.

Provide opportunities for exploration: Create a safe and stimulating environment where your baby can explore and interact with their surroundings. Offer age-appropriate toys, sensory experiences, and outdoor play opportunities to encourage curiosity and discovery.

Model positive social behaviors: Be a positive role model for your baby by demonstrating kindness, empathy, and respect in your interactions with others. Show appreciation for diversity and inclusivity, and celebrate the unique qualities and strengths of each individual.

By fostering positive social interactions and modeling healthy relationship dynamics, you can help your baby develop the social skills and emotional intelligence they need to thrive in a complex and interconnected world.

Chapter 3

Cognitive Stimulation

Cognitive stimulation is essential for your baby's intellectual development, laying the groundwork for critical thinking, problem-solving, and lifelong learning. In this chapter, we will explore the importance of early learning and brain development, stimulating activities for cognitive growth, and creating an enriched learning environment that fosters curiosity, exploration, and discovery.

Early Learning and Brain Development

The first few years of life are a critical period for brain development, with billions of neural connections forming and shaping the foundation for future learning and cognitive abilities. During this time, your baby's brain is highly plastic and responsive to environmental stimuli, making it an opportune time to nurture cognitive development through enriching experiences and interactions.

Research has shown that early experiences play a significant role in shaping brain development, with positive interactions and stimulating environments contributing to enhanced cognitive abilities later in life. By providing your baby with a rich and varied array of experiences, you can help support their cognitive growth and lay the foundation for a lifetime of learning.

Some key principles to keep in mind when fostering early learning and brain development include:

Responsive caregiving: Engage in responsive caregiving practices that support your baby's exploration, curiosity, and learning. Respond promptly and sensitively to your baby's cues and signals, providing encouragement, praise, and support as they navigate the world around them.

Stimulating environments: Create an environment that is rich in sensory experiences and opportunities for exploration. Offer age-appropriate toys, books, and games that stimulate your baby's senses and encourage them to engage with their surroundings.

Language exposure: Expose your baby to a rich and varied language environment, including spoken language, music, and storytelling. Engage in frequent conversations, sing songs, and read books together to promote language development and cognitive growth.

Encouragement of curiosity: Encourage your baby's natural curiosity and desire to explore by providing opportunities for hands-on learning and discovery. Offer open-ended toys and materials that allow for creative and imaginative play, and support your baby's exploration of their environment with enthusiasm and encouragement.

Promotion of independence: Foster your baby's growing sense of autonomy and independence by allowing them to explore and experiment with their environment in safe and supervised ways. Offer support and guidance as needed, but allow your baby the freedom to discover and learn at their own pace.

By prioritizing responsive caregiving, stimulating environments, language exposure, encouragement of curiosity, and promotion of independence, you can help support your baby's cognitive development and lay the foundation for a lifetime of learning and intellectual growth.

Stimulating Activities for Cognitive Growth

Engaging in stimulating activities is an effective way to promote cognitive growth and development in your baby. By providing opportunities for exploration, problem-solving, and creative expression, you can help stimulate your baby's curiosity, foster critical thinking skills, and encourage intellectual growth.

Some stimulating activities to consider include:

Sensory play: Sensory play activities engage your baby's senses and promote exploration and discovery. Offer materials such as water, sand, playdough, and textured fabrics for your baby to explore through touch, sight, and sound.

Puzzle play: Age-appropriate puzzles and shape sorters can help your baby develop problem-solving skills, spatial awareness, and hand-eye coordination. Start with simple puzzles and gradually increase the complexity as your baby's skills develop.

Exploratory play: Provide opportunities for exploratory play by offering toys and materials that encourage investigation and manipulation. Allow your baby to experiment with cause and effect, patterns, and relationships as they explore their environment.

Imaginative play: Encourage imaginative play by providing open-ended toys and props that inspire creativity and storytelling. Offer dress-up clothes, puppets, dolls, and toy vehicles that allow your baby to engage in imaginative role-play and storytelling.

Music and movement: Music and movement activities stimulate multiple areas of the brain and promote cognitive development. Sing songs, play musical instruments, and engage in movement activities such as dancing, clapping, and marching to promote rhythm, coordination, and auditory processing skills.

Nature exploration: Spend time outdoors exploring nature and the natural world with your baby. Take nature walks, visit parks and playgrounds, and engage in activities such as gardening, birdwatching, and collecting natural objects to promote curiosity, observation skills, and appreciation for the environment.

By incorporating stimulating activities into your daily routine, you can provide your baby with the rich and varied experiences they need to support cognitive growth and development. Remember to follow your baby's lead, offering support and encouragement as they explore and learn at their own pace.

Creating an Enriched Learning Environment

Creating an enriched learning environment is key to fostering cognitive development and promoting intellectual growth in your baby. By surrounding your baby with stimulating materials, engaging experiences, and supportive interactions, you can create a nurturing environment that encourages curiosity, exploration, and discovery.

Some strategies for creating an enriched learning environment include:

Provide a variety of learning materials: Offer a diverse range of toys, books, and materials that stimulate your baby's senses and promote exploration and creativity. Include toys that encourage problem-solving, imaginative play, and fine motor skills development.

Designate play spaces: Create designated play areas within your home where your baby can explore and engage in stimulating activities. Ensure these spaces are safe, comfortable, and free from distractions, allowing your baby to focus and concentrate on their play.

Rotate toys and materials: Rotate toys and materials regularly to keep your baby's environment fresh and engaging. Introduce new toys, books, and activities periodically to provide novel experiences and opportunities for learning and discovery.

Promote open-ended play: Offer toys and materials that can be used in multiple ways, encouraging open-ended play and creative expression. Avoid toys that are overly prescriptive or limit your baby's imagination, and instead focus on toys that promote exploration, problem-solving, and imaginative play.

Engage in meaningful interactions: Interact with your baby in meaningful and responsive ways that support their cognitive development. Engage in conversations, sing songs, and read books together to promote language development and stimulate intellectual growth.

Encourage exploration and curiosity: Encourage your baby's natural curiosity and desire to explore by providing opportunities for hands-on learning and discovery. Offer materials that encourage sensory exploration, experimentation, and problem-solving, and support your baby's exploration with enthusiasm and encouragement.

By creating an enriched learning environment that is rich in stimulating materials, engaging experiences, and supportive interactions, you can foster cognitive development and promote intellectual growth in your baby. Remember to follow your baby's interests and cues, providing support and encouragement as they explore and learn at their own pace.

Chapter 4

Communication

Communication is the cornerstone of your relationship with your baby, facilitating connection, understanding, and emotional bonding. In this chapter, we will explore the various aspects of communication between parents and babies, including understanding baby's cries and vocalizations, building language skills through interaction, and the importance of non-verbal communication in fostering bonding and connection.

Understanding Baby's Cries and Vocalizations

Crying is your baby's primary means of communication, signaling a variety of needs and emotions, from hunger and discomfort to fatigue and overstimulation. Understanding your baby's cries and vocalizations is essential for meeting their needs and providing the support and comfort they require.

While it can be challenging to decipher the meaning behind your baby's cries, there are some common cues and signals to watch for:

Hunger: Hunger is one of the most common reasons for crying in babies. Look for early hunger cues such as sucking on fists or rooting movements, and offer feeding promptly to satisfy your baby's hunger.

Discomfort: Your baby may cry if they are uncomfortable due to factors such as a wet or soiled diaper, tight clothing, or being too hot or cold. Check for any obvious sources of discomfort and address them promptly to provide relief.

Fatigue: Babies may become fussy or irritable when they are tired or overstimulated. Look for yawning, rubbing eyes, or becoming increasingly fussy as signs that your baby may need rest and quiet time.

Overstimulation: Too much noise, activity, or stimulation can overwhelm your baby and lead to crying. Pay attention to your baby's cues and provide a calm and soothing environment when they become overstimulated.

Discomfort or pain: Your baby may cry if they are experiencing discomfort or pain, such as from gas, colic, or teething. Comfort and soothe your baby, and consult with your pediatrician if you suspect they may be in pain.

In addition to crying, your baby will also communicate through vocalizations such as cooing, babbling, and laughter. These early vocalizations are an important precursor to language development, signaling your baby's growing ability to communicate and engage with the world around them.

Building Language Skills Through Interaction

Language development begins long before your baby says their first words, with babies actively listening and absorbing language from the moment they are born. By engaging in interactive and responsive communication with your baby, you can help support their language development and lay the foundation for effective communication skills.

Some strategies for building language skills through interaction include:

Talking to your baby: Engage in frequent conversations with your baby, describing your activities, narrating your day, and sharing your thoughts and feelings. Use simple, repetitive language and a warm and expressive tone to capture your baby's attention and promote language development.

Reading together: Reading to your baby is one of the most effective ways to promote language development and literacy skills. Choose age-appropriate board books with colorful illustrations and simple text, and make reading together a part of your daily routine.

Singing songs and nursery rhymes: Singing songs and reciting nursery rhymes exposes your baby to rhythm, melody, and language patterns, helping to promote phonological awareness and language development. Choose familiar songs and rhymes and sing them with enthusiasm and expression.

Responding to your baby's vocalizations: Encourage your baby's early vocalizations by responding with enthusiasm and attention. Mirror your baby's sounds, gestures, and facial expressions, and engage in back-and-forth exchanges that mimic the give-and-take of conversation.

Using gestures and signs: Incorporate gestures and signs into your communication with your baby to support language development and comprehension. Use simple signs such as "more," "all done," and "please" to enhance your baby's understanding and facilitate communication.

By engaging in interactive and responsive communication with your baby, you can help support their language development and lay the foundation for effective communication skills that will serve them throughout their lives.

Non-Verbal Communication and Bonding

Non-verbal communication, including facial expressions, gestures, and body language, plays a crucial role in fostering bonding and connection between parents and babies. From the moment they are born, babies are attuned to their caregivers' non-verbal cues, using them to interpret and respond to the world around them.

Some ways to enhance non-verbal communication and bonding with your baby include:

Eye contact: Make frequent eye contact with your baby during interactions, signaling your attentiveness and engagement. Eye contact helps establish a connection and promotes feelings of security and trust between you and your baby.

Facial expressions: Use facial expressions such as smiles, frowns, and raised eyebrows to convey emotions and communicate with your baby. Smile and make eye contact when your baby smiles or vocalizes, reinforcing their positive behavior and fostering emotional connection.

Touch: Physical touch is a powerful way to communicate love and affection to your baby. Cuddle, hold, and gently stroke your baby to provide comfort and reassurance, and engage in skin-to-skin contact to promote bonding and attachment.

Gentle vocalizations: Use soothing and comforting vocalizations such as cooing, humming, and gentle singing to communicate with your baby. Your tone of voice can convey warmth, reassurance, and emotional support, helping to strengthen the bond between you and your baby.

Responsive interactions: Be responsive to your baby's cues and signals, adjusting your interactions and responses based on their needs and preferences. By tuning into your baby's non-verbal communication, you can foster a sense of security and trust, promoting healthy attachment and bonding.

By incorporating non-verbal communication into your interactions with your baby, you can strengthen the bond between you and promote emotional connection and well-being.

Chapter 5

Health and Wellness

Ensuring the health and wellness of your baby is paramount to their overall development and happiness. In this chapter, we will delve into key aspects of infant health and wellness, including the importance of following an immunization schedule and preventive care, recognizing common health concerns and knowing when to seek help, and nurturing a healthy lifestyle that promotes optimal well-being.

Immunization Schedule and Preventive Car

Following an immunization schedule and implementing preventive care measures are essential components of safeguarding your baby's health and protecting them from preventable diseases. Immunizations are critical for building immunity against serious illnesses and reducing the risk of outbreaks within the community.

It is essential to work closely with your pediatrician to ensure your baby receives all recommended vaccinations according to the schedule outlined by leading health authorities, such as the Centers for Disease Control and Prevention (CDC) and the World Health Organization (WHO). The recommended immunization schedule typically begins shortly after birth and continues through early childhood, with vaccines administered at specific ages to provide optimal protection.

Common vaccines administered during infancy include those for diseases such as:

Hepatitis B

Polio

Diphtheria, tetanus, and pertussis (DTaP)

Haemophilus influenzae type b (Hib)

Pneumococcal conjugate (PCV)

Rotavirus

Measles, mumps, and rubella (MMR)

In addition to following the immunization schedule, implementing preventive care measures can help keep your baby healthy and reduce the risk of illness. Some preventive care practices to consider include:

Breastfeeding: Breastfeeding provides numerous health benefits for both you and your baby, including immune system support and protection against infections. Aim to breastfeed exclusively for the first six months of life, and continue breastfeeding alongside complementary foods for up to two years or longer.

Good hygiene practices: Practice good hygiene to prevent the spread of germs and reduce the risk of illness. Wash your hands frequently, especially before handling your baby or preparing food, and teach older siblings and family members to do the same. Keep your baby's environment clean and sanitized, paying special attention to commonly-touched surfaces and objects.

Regular check-ups: Schedule regular well-baby check-ups with your pediatrician to monitor your baby's growth and development, track milestones, and address any concerns or questions you may have. Well-baby visits typically include physical exams, developmental screenings, and discussions about nutrition, safety, and immunizations.

By following the recommended immunization schedule and implementing preventive care measures, you can help protect your baby from serious illnesses and promote their overall health and well-being.

Common Health Concerns and When to Seek Help

Despite your best efforts to keep your baby healthy, it is common for infants to experience occasional health concerns and minor ailments. While many of these issues are normal and resolve on their own, some may require medical attention. It is essential to be aware of common health concerns in infancy and know when to seek help from your pediatrician.

Some common health concerns in infancy include:

Fevers: Fevers are a common symptom of illness in babies and are typically a sign that the body is fighting off an infection. While low-grade fevers are usually harmless and may resolve on their own, high fevers or fevers accompanied by other concerning symptoms should prompt a call to your pediatrician.

Respiratory infections: Babies are susceptible to respiratory infections such as colds, flu, and respiratory syncytial virus (RSV). Symptoms may include coughing, congestion, fever, and difficulty breathing. Seek medical attention if your baby's symptoms are severe or persistent, or if they develop signs of respiratory distress.

Gastrointestinal issues: Babies may experience digestive issues such as reflux, colic, or constipation, which can cause discomfort and distress. While some degree of spitting up, gas, and fussiness is normal, persistent or severe symptoms may warrant evaluation by your pediatrician.

Skin conditions: Skin conditions such as diaper rash, eczema, and cradle cap are common in infancy and are usually mild and self-limiting. However, persistent or severe skin issues may require treatment or management by a healthcare provider.

Developmental concerns: Keep an eye on your baby's developmental milestones and consult with your pediatrician if you have concerns about their progress. Early intervention is key for addressing developmental delays or concerns and ensuring your baby receives the support they need.

It is essential to trust your instincts as a parent and seek help if you have concerns about your baby's health or well-being. Never hesitate to contact your pediatrician if you are unsure whether your baby's symptoms warrant medical attention.

Nurturing a Healthy Lifestyle

Nurturing a healthy lifestyle is crucial for promoting optimal health and wellness in your baby. By prioritizing nutrition, physical activity, sleep, and emotional well-being, you can help support your baby's overall development and lay the foundation for a lifetime of healthy habits.

Some strategies for nurturing a healthy lifestyle in infancy include:

Nutrition: Offer a balanced diet that includes a variety of nutrient-rich foods to support your baby's growth and development. Breastfeed exclusively for the first six months of life, and introduce complementary foods alongside continued breastfeeding starting around six months of age. Offer a variety of fruits, vegetables, whole grains, lean proteins, and healthy fats, and avoid introducing foods that are high in sugar, salt, or artificial additives.

Physical activity: Encourage daily physical activity and playtime to support your baby's physical development and motor skills. Provide opportunities for tummy time, floor play, and supervised exploration to help your baby build strength, coordination, and balance.

Sleep: Establish healthy sleep habits and routines to ensure your baby gets adequate rest and quality sleep. Create a calming bedtime routine that signals to your baby that it's time to sleep, and provide a safe and comfortable sleep environment free from distractions and hazards.

Emotional well-being: Prioritize your baby's emotional well-being by providing a nurturing and responsive caregiving environment. Offer plenty of love, affection, and attention, and respond promptly and sensitively to your baby's cues and signals. Create a supportive and predictable routine that helps your baby feel safe, secure, and loved.

Limit screen time: Minimize your baby's exposure to screens and electronic devices, as excessive screen time can interfere with sleep, physical activity, and cognitive development. Instead, encourage hands-on play, exploration, and interaction with the world around them.

By prioritizing nutrition, physical activity, sleep, and emotional well-being, you can help promote optimal health and wellness in your baby and lay the foundation for a lifetime of healthy habits.

Chapter 6

Sleep Solutions

Adequate sleep is essential for your baby's health, development, and overall well-being. In this chapter, we will explore strategies for establishing healthy sleep habits, addressing common sleep challenges, and implementing sleep safety guidelines to ensure your baby sleeps soundly and safely.

Establishing Healthy Sleep Habits

Establishing healthy sleep habits is crucial for promoting restful and rejuvenating sleep for your baby. By creating a consistent bedtime routine, providing a conducive sleep environment, and promoting good sleep hygiene practices, you can help set the stage for restful nights and well-rested days.

Some strategies for establishing healthy sleep habits include:

Consistent bedtime routine: Establish a calming bedtime routine that signals to your baby that it's time to wind down and prepare for sleep. Aim to start the bedtime routine around the same time each night and include activities such as a warm bath, gentle massage, bedtime story, or lullabies to help your baby relax and transition to sleep.

Create a conducive sleep environment: Create a sleep environment that is quiet, dark, and comfortable to promote restful sleep. Use blackout curtains or shades to block out light, maintain a comfortable room temperature, and remove any potential sources of noise or distractions that may disrupt your baby's sleep.

Promote self-soothing skills: Encourage your baby to develop self-soothing skills that enable them to fall asleep independently and self-settle during nighttime awakenings. Offer comfort and reassurance as needed, but gradually encourage your baby to learn to soothe themselves back to sleep without relying on external interventions.

Establish a consistent sleep schedule: Establish a consistent sleep schedule that includes regular nap times and bedtime, based on your baby's age and developmental stage. Consistency is key for helping your baby regulate their sleep-wake cycle and establish healthy sleep patterns.

Monitor sleep cues: Pay attention to your baby's sleep cues and signals, such as rubbing eyes, yawning, or becoming fussy, and respond promptly to their sleep needs. By responding to your baby's cues in a timely manner, you can help prevent overtiredness and promote restful sleep.

By implementing these strategies consistently and persistently, you can help establish healthy sleep habits that support your baby's physical, cognitive, and emotional well-being.

Addressing Sleep Challenges

Despite your best efforts to establish healthy sleep habits, it is common for babies to experience sleep challenges at various stages of development. From difficulty falling asleep to frequent nighttime awakenings, sleep challenges can be stressful for both you and your baby. However, with patience, consistency, and support, many sleep challenges can be successfully addressed.

Some common sleep challenges and strategies for addressing them include:

Difficulty falling asleep: If your baby has difficulty falling asleep, consider adjusting their bedtime routine to include calming activities that promote relaxation, such as gentle massage, rocking, or soothing music. Avoid stimulating activities or screens before bedtime, as they can interfere with your baby's ability to fall asleep.

Frequent nighttime awakenings: Nighttime awakenings are common in infancy and are often due to factors such as hunger, discomfort, or developmental milestones. If your baby wakes up frequently during the night, try to respond promptly to their needs while also encouraging them to self-soothe and fall back asleep independently.

Short naps: Some babies struggle to take long or restful naps during the day, leading to overtiredness and irritability. To encourage longer naps, create a conducive sleep environment, establish a consistent nap schedule, and offer comfort and reassurance as needed. Gradually extend nap times by gradually adjusting your baby's sleep routine and schedule.

Nighttime feeding: If your baby relies on nighttime feedings for comfort or nourishment, consider gradually reducing the frequency of feedings and encouraging your baby to consume more calories during the day. Offer additional feedings or larger meals before bedtime to help satisfy your baby's hunger and promote longer stretches of sleep at night.

Separation anxiety: As babies grow and develop, they may experience separation anxiety, making it difficult for them to settle and sleep independently. Offer comfort and reassurance as needed, and gradually encourage your baby to become more comfortable with separation by gradually increasing the distance between you during bedtime routines.

By addressing sleep challenges with patience, consistency, and support, you can help your baby develop healthy sleep habits and enjoy restful nights and well-rested days.

Sleep Safety Guidelines

Ensuring your baby's safety during sleep is paramount to reducing the risk of sudden infant death syndrome (SIDS) and other sleep-related accidents. By following sleep safety guidelines recommended by pediatricians and health authorities, you can create a safe sleep environment that promotes peace of mind and protects your baby from harm.

Some sleep safety guidelines to consider include:

Back to sleep: Always place your baby on their back to sleep, both for naps and nighttime sleep. This position reduces the risk of SIDS and allows your baby to breathe more freely.

Use a firm sleep surface: Provide your baby with a firm and flat sleep surface, such as a crib, bassinet, or portable crib mattress, that meets current safety standards. Avoid soft bedding, pillows, stuffed animals, and other loose objects that could pose a suffocation hazard.

Keep the sleep environment clear: Keep the sleep environment clear of clutter, toys, blankets, and other items that could obstruct your baby's breathing or pose a suffocation risk. Use a fitted sheet to cover the mattress, and dress your baby in lightweight sleep clothing to prevent overheating.

Room-sharing without bed-sharing: Room-sharing with your baby, where your baby sleeps in a separate sleep space in the same room as you, is recommended for the first six to twelve months of life. However, avoid bed-sharing with your baby, as it increases the risk of SIDS and other sleep-related accidents.

Avoid overheating: Keep the room temperature comfortable and avoid overdressing your baby or overdressing the sleep environment, as overheating increases the risk of SIDS. Aim for a room temperature between 68°F and 72°F and dress your baby in light, breathable sleep clothing.

Offer a pacifier at bedtime: Consider offering a pacifier at bedtime, as it has been shown to reduce the risk of SIDS. However, wait until breastfeeding is well established before introducing a pacifier, usually around three to four weeks of age.

By following these sleep safety guidelines consistently and diligently, you can create a safe sleep environment for your baby and reduce the risk of sleep-related accidents and SIDS.

Chapter 7

Balancing Work and Parenting

Balancing the demands of work and parenting can be challenging, but with careful planning, support, and flexibility, it is possible to thrive in both roles. In this chapter, we will explore strategies for working parents to effectively manage their professional responsibilities while nurturing their relationships with their children, maintaining work-life balance, and creating supportive networks that help alleviate the pressures of juggling work and parenting.

Strategies for Working Parents

As a working parent, it is essential to develop strategies that enable you to fulfill your professional obligations while also meeting the needs of your family. By prioritizing time management, setting realistic expectations, and establishing boundaries, you can create a framework that supports both your career and your role as a parent.

Some strategies for working parents to consider include:

Establish clear priorities: Identify your top priorities both at work and at home and allocate your time and energy accordingly. Determine what tasks and activities are essential to your professional success and focus on those during designated work hours, while also making time for quality family time and self-care.

Maximize efficiency: Find ways to streamline your work processes and maximize efficiency to make the most of your time. Use tools and technology to automate repetitive tasks, prioritize your workload based on urgency and importance, and delegate tasks when appropriate to free up time for higher-value activities.

Set boundaries: Establish clear boundaries between work and home life to prevent burnout and maintain balance. Define specific work hours and designate dedicated time for family activities and personal pursuits, and communicate these boundaries to your employer, colleagues, and family members.

Practice time management: Implement time management techniques such as prioritizing tasks, setting deadlines, and using calendars and planners to stay organized and on track. Break larger tasks into smaller, manageable steps and allocate time each day for focused work, family time, and relaxation.

Flexibility and adaptability: Embrace flexibility and adaptability to accommodate the changing demands of work and parenting. Recognize that unforeseen challenges and disruptions may arise, and be prepared to adjust your plans and priorities as needed to meet the needs of both your career and your family.

By implementing these strategies consistently and proactively, you can effectively navigate the complexities of balancing work and parenting and create a fulfilling and rewarding experience for yourself and your family.

Maintaining Work-Life Balance

Maintaining a healthy work-life balance is essential for the well-being of working parents and their families. By prioritizing self-care, setting boundaries, and fostering meaningful connections with loved ones, you can achieve greater harmony between your professional and personal lives and experience greater satisfaction and fulfillment in both realms.

Some strategies for maintaining work-life balance as a working parent include:

Prioritize self-care: Make time for self-care activities that recharge your physical, mental, and emotional batteries. Prioritize activities that bring you joy and relaxation, such as exercise, hobbies, meditation, or spending time outdoors, and schedule regular self-care breaks into your routine.

Set boundaries: Establish clear boundaries between work and personal time to prevent burnout and maintain balance. Communicate your availability and expectations to your employer and colleagues, and resist the temptation to constantly check emails or take work calls outside of designated work hours.

Spend quality time with family: Prioritize quality time with your family by scheduling regular activities and outings that allow you to connect and bond with your loved ones. Make family meals, game nights, and outdoor adventures a priority, and be fully present and engaged during these moments together.

Delegate and outsource tasks: Delegate household tasks and responsibilities to family members, partners, or hired help to lighten your workload and free up time for more meaningful activities. Consider outsourcing tasks such as cleaning, cooking, or childcare to reduce stress and create more time for relaxation and family time.

Practice mindfulness: Cultivate mindfulness and presence in your daily life by focusing on the present moment and embracing gratitude and appreciation for the blessings in your life. Practice mindfulness techniques such as meditation, deep breathing, or journaling to reduce stress and enhance overall well-being.

By prioritizing self-care, setting boundaries, and fostering meaningful connections with loved ones, you can maintain a healthy work-life balance and experience greater fulfillment and happiness in both your professional and personal life.

Creating Supportive Networks

Building a supportive network of family, friends, colleagues, and fellow parents can be invaluable for working parents as they navigate the challenges of balancing work and parenting. By surrounding yourself with supportive individuals who understand your unique circumstances and offer encouragement, advice, and practical assistance, you can feel more confident and capable in managing the demands of both roles.

Some ways to create supportive networks as a working parent include:

Join parent groups and communities: Seek out parent groups, support networks, and online communities where you can connect with other working parents who share similar experiences and challenges. Participate in parenting forums, social media groups, or local meetups to share advice, resources, and camaraderie with fellow parents.

Lean on family and friends: Reach out to family members and friends for support and assistance with childcare, household tasks, or emotional support when needed. Build a network of trusted individuals who can offer help and encouragement during busy or stressful times.

Connect with colleagues: Forge connections with colleagues who are also working parents and share strategies, tips, and resources for balancing work and parenting responsibilities. Establish a supportive work culture that recognizes and accommodates the needs of working parents, such as flexible work arrangements or family-friendly policies.

Seek professional support: Consider seeking professional support from therapists, counselors, or coaches who specialize in work-life balance, parenting, or stress management. A professional can offer personalized guidance, strategies, and tools to help you navigate the challenges of balancing work and parenting and enhance your overall well-being.

Practice reciprocity: Offer support and assistance to other working parents in your network, reciprocating the kindness and generosity you receive from others. By building a culture of mutual support and reciprocity, you can create a strong and resilient community that benefits everyone involved.

By creating supportive networks of family, friends, colleagues, and fellow parents, you can find encouragement, guidance, and practical assistance as you navigate the complexities of balancing work and parenting.

Chapter 8

Financial Planning for Parenthood

Financial planning is a crucial aspect of preparing for parenthood, as it allows you to anticipate and manage the costs associated with raising a child, while also setting the stage for your family's long-term financial security and stability. In this chapter, we will explore strategies for budgeting for your baby's needs, investing in your child's future, and implementing smart financial strategies that support your family's financial well-being.

Budgeting for Baby's Needs

Budgeting for your baby's needs involves identifying and prioritizing expenses related to childcare, healthcare, education, and daily living, and allocating your financial resources accordingly. By creating a comprehensive budget that accounts for both fixed and variable expenses, you can ensure that you have the financial means to provide for your baby's needs while also maintaining your own financial stability.

Some key expenses to consider when budgeting for your baby's needs include:

Childcare: Childcare costs can vary significantly depending on factors such as location, type of care (e.g., daycare, nanny, family care), and your child's age. Research childcare options in your area, compare costs, and budget accordingly to ensure that you can afford quality care for your baby.

Healthcare: Healthcare expenses for your baby may include medical appointments, vaccinations, prescriptions, and health insurance premiums. Review your health insurance coverage to understand what is covered and what out-of-pocket costs you may be responsible for, and budget accordingly for healthcare expenses.

Diapers and supplies: Diapers, wipes, formula (if applicable), and other baby supplies can add up quickly. Estimate your monthly expenses for these items and budget accordingly to ensure that you have an adequate supply on hand at all times.

Clothing and gear: Babies grow quickly and may require new clothing and gear as they outgrow their old items. Budget for regular purchases of clothing, shoes, and gear such as strollers, car seats, cribs, and high chairs to accommodate your baby's changing needs.

Education and enrichment: While it may seem premature, it's never too early to start saving for your child's education. Consider opening a college savings account such as a 529 plan or a custodial account and contribute regularly to help cover future education expenses.

Daily living expenses: Don't forget to budget for everyday expenses such as groceries, utilities, transportation, and household expenses. Review your current spending habits and identify areas where you can cut back or reallocate funds to accommodate your baby's needs.

By creating a comprehensive budget that accounts for all of your baby's needs, you can ensure that you have the financial means to provide for your child's well-being and development while also maintaining your own financial stability.

Investing in Your Child's Future

Investing in your child's future involves setting aside funds for their education, healthcare, and other long-term needs, while also teaching them the value of financial responsibility and independence. By starting early and adopting a disciplined approach to saving and investing, you can build a solid financial foundation that supports your child's growth and development over time.

Some strategies for investing in your child's future include:

Start a college savings plan: Consider opening a college savings account such as a 529 plan, which offers tax-advantaged savings for educational expenses. Contribute regularly to the plan and explore investment options that align with your risk tolerance and investment goals.

Teach financial literacy: Educate your child about the importance of saving, budgeting, and investing from an early age. Involve them in household budgeting discussions, encourage them to set savings goals, and provide opportunities for them to earn and manage their own money.

Invest in a diversified portfolio: Consider investing in a diversified portfolio of stocks, bonds, and other assets to help grow your child's savings over time. Consult with a financial advisor to develop an investment strategy that aligns with your goals and risk tolerance.

Explore insurance options: Consider purchasing life insurance or disability insurance to protect your child's financial future in the event of unforeseen circumstances. Research different insurance options and select coverage that provides adequate protection for your family's needs.

Encourage entrepreneurial spirit: Foster your child's entrepreneurial spirit by encouraging them to explore business opportunities, develop creative ideas, and take calculated risks. Teach them about entrepreneurship, innovation, and financial management, and provide support and guidance as they pursue their goals.

By investing in your child's future through education savings, financial literacy, diversified investments, insurance protection, and entrepreneurial opportunities, you can help set them on a path to financial security and success.

Smart Financial Strategies

In addition to budgeting for your baby's needs and investing in their future, implementing smart financial strategies can help you make the most of your resources and achieve your financial goals as a parent. By prioritizing savings, managing debt, and planning for emergencies, you can build financial resilience and security for your family.

Some smart financial strategies for parents to consider include:

Build an emergency fund: Set aside funds in an emergency savings account to cover unexpected expenses such as medical bills, car repairs, or job loss. Aim to save three to six months' worth of living expenses to provide a financial cushion in case of emergencies.

Pay off high-interest debt: Prioritize paying off high-interest debt such as credit card debt or personal loans to reduce interest costs and free up funds for other financial goals. Consider consolidating debt or negotiating lower interest rates to accelerate debt repayment and improve your financial health.

Automate savings: Set up automatic transfers from your checking account to your savings or investment accounts to automate your savings and ensure consistent contributions over time. Pay yourself first by prioritizing savings goals and treating them as non-negotiable expenses.

Review and adjust your budget regularly: Review your budget regularly to track your spending, identify areas for improvement, and adjust your budget as needed to align with your financial goals. Be flexible and willing to make changes as your family's needs and circumstances evolve.

Seek professional advice: Consider seeking advice from a financial advisor or planner who can provide personalized guidance and recommendations based on your financial goals and circumstances. A professional can help you develop a comprehensive financial plan, identify opportunities for growth, and navigate complex financial decisions.

By implementing these smart financial strategies, you can build financial resilience, achieve your financial goals, and provide a secure and stable future for your family.

Chapter 9

Sibling Dynamics

Sibling relationships play a significant role in shaping a child's social and emotional development. From preparing your child for the arrival of a new sibling to fostering positive sibling relationships and addressing sibling rivalry, understanding and navigating sibling dynamics is essential for promoting harmony and cohesion within the family unit. In this chapter, we will explore strategies for preparing your child for a sibling, fostering positive sibling relationships, and addressing sibling rivalry with empathy and understanding.

Preparing Your Child for a Sibling

Introducing a new sibling into the family can be both exciting and challenging for older children. To help your child prepare for the arrival of a new sibling, it is essential to involve them in the process, address their concerns and anxieties, and foster a sense of excitement and anticipation about becoming a big brother or sister.

Some strategies for preparing your child for a sibling include:

Start early: Begin preparing your child for the arrival of a new sibling as soon as possible, ideally during the pregnancy. Share the news with your child in an age-appropriate way, and involve them in discussions and preparations for the new baby.

Read books and stories: Read books and stories about new siblings and families to your child to help them understand what to expect and normalize the experience of welcoming a new baby into the family. Choose books that depict positive sibling relationships and emphasize the joys of being a big brother or sister.

Involve your child: Involve your child in preparations for the new baby, such as choosing baby names, decorating the nursery, and selecting baby clothes and toys. Encourage your child to express their feelings and opinions about the upcoming changes and reassure them that their role as a big sibling is important and valued.

Practice empathy and understanding: Be mindful of your child's feelings and emotions about the arrival of a new sibling, and validate their concerns and anxieties with empathy and understanding. Reassure your child that it's normal to feel a mix of emotions about the changes ahead and provide opportunities for them to express their feelings openly and honestly.

Establish routines and traditions: Establish special routines and traditions that involve your child in caring for and bonding with the new baby, such as reading bedtime stories together, taking turns feeding or changing diapers, or going on family outings and adventures. Create opportunities for your child to feel included and valued as a member of the growing family.

By involving your child in preparations for the new sibling, addressing their concerns and anxieties with empathy and understanding, and establishing special routines and traditions that promote bonding and connection, you can help prepare your child for the arrival of a new sibling with confidence and excitement.

Fostering Positive Sibling Relationships

Fostering positive sibling relationships is essential for promoting harmony and cohesion within the family unit. By cultivating a supportive and nurturing environment that encourages cooperation, communication, and empathy, you can help your children develop strong and resilient sibling bonds that last a lifetime.

Some strategies for fostering positive sibling relationships include:

Encourage cooperation and teamwork: Encourage your children to work together and cooperate on tasks and activities, such as cleaning up toys, completing chores, or playing games. Emphasize the importance of teamwork and collaboration, and praise and reward positive interactions and efforts to help each other.

Promote communication and problem-solving: Teach your children effective communication and problem-solving skills to help them navigate conflicts and disagreements constructively. Encourage them to express their feelings and perspectives openly and respectfully, and guide them in finding mutually agreeable solutions to conflicts and disputes.

Create opportunities for bonding: Create opportunities for your children to bond and connect with each other through shared activities and experiences. Plan family outings, game nights, or special outings that allow siblings to spend quality time together and build memories and traditions that strengthen their bond.

Celebrate individual strengths and interests: Celebrate and affirm each child's unique strengths, talents, and interests, and encourage them to support and celebrate each other's achievements and accomplishments. Emphasize the importance of kindness, generosity, and mutual respect in sibling relationships, and model these values in your interactions with your children.

Set a positive example: Be a positive role model for your children by demonstrating healthy and respectful relationships in your own interactions with family members and others. Show appreciation for your children's efforts to support and care for each other, and praise and encourage positive behavior and acts of kindness.

By fostering cooperation, communication, empathy, and mutual respect within the family, you can help your children develop strong and positive sibling relationships that enrich their lives and contribute to their overall well-being.

Addressing Sibling Rivalry

Sibling rivalry is a common and natural part of sibling relationships, but it can also be a source of stress and conflict within the family. By understanding the underlying causes of sibling rivalry and implementing strategies to address conflicts and promote harmony, you can help your children navigate their differences and develop healthier and more resilient relationships with each other.

Some strategies for addressing sibling rivalry include:

Acknowledge and validate feelings: Acknowledge and validate your children's feelings and emotions about sibling rivalry with empathy and understanding. Help them identify and express their feelings openly and constructively, and reassure them that it's normal to experience jealousy, frustration, or anger at times.

Set clear expectations and boundaries: Set clear expectations and boundaries for acceptable behavior and conflict resolution within the family, and enforce consequences for disrespectful or harmful behavior. Encourage your children to communicate their needs and concerns respectfully and to seek help from you or another trusted adult when conflicts arise.

Promote fairness and equity: Promote fairness and equity in your interactions with your children and avoid comparing them or playing favorites. Treat each child as an individual with unique needs and preferences, and avoid making judgments or assumptions based on stereotypes or preconceptions.

Encourage empathy and perspective-taking: Encourage your children to empathize with each other's perspectives and to consider how their words and actions impact their siblings. Teach them to take turns listening and speaking, and to seek compromise and resolution rather than escalating conflicts.

Provide opportunities for one-on-one time: Provide each child with individual attention and one-on-one time with you and other family members to strengthen their bond and reduce feelings of rivalry or competition. Plan special outings or activities that allow each child to feel valued and appreciated as an individual.

By addressing sibling rivalry with empathy, understanding, and proactive strategies for conflict resolution, you can help your children navigate their differences and develop healthier and more harmonious relationships with each other.

Chapter 10

Self-Care for Parents

Parenting is a demanding and rewarding journey that requires dedication, patience, and love. However, amidst the responsibilities of caring for your children, it's essential not to overlook your own well-being. Taking care of yourself is not selfish; it's necessary for you to be the best parent you can be. In this chapter, we'll explore the importance of self-care for parents, strategies for finding time for yourself, and the benefits of seeking support and building resilience.

The Importance of Self-Care

Self-care is more than just pampering yourself; it's about prioritizing your physical, mental, and emotional health to maintain balance and prevent burnout. As a parent, practicing self-care is essential for your overall well-being and your ability to care for your children effectively. Here's why self-care is important:

Stress management: Parenting can be stressful, and chronic stress can take a toll on your physical and mental health. Practicing self-care techniques such as mindfulness, relaxation exercises, and hobbies can help reduce stress levels and promote a sense of calm and well-being.

Modeling healthy behavior: Children learn by example, and by prioritizing self-care, you're modeling healthy behavior and teaching your children the importance of taking care of themselves. By demonstrating self-compassion and self-care practices, you're instilling valuable life skills in your children.

Enhanced resilience: Taking care of yourself strengthens your resilience, allowing you to bounce back from challenges and setbacks more effectively. When you prioritize self-care, you're better equipped to handle the ups and downs of parenting with grace and resilience.

Improved physical health: Self-care practices such as regular exercise, nutritious eating, and adequate sleep contribute to better physical health, giving you the energy and vitality you need to keep up with the demands of parenting.

Enhanced mental health: Self-care is crucial for maintaining good mental health and preventing burnout, anxiety, and depression. Taking time for activities that bring you joy and fulfillment can boost your mood and overall mental well-being.

Finding Time for Yourself

Finding time for yourself as a parent can be challenging, but it's essential for your well-being. Here are some strategies for carving out time for self-care:

Schedule self-care: Treat self-care activities as non-negotiable appointments in your calendar. Block out time each day or week for activities that recharge you, whether it's exercise, meditation, reading, or hobbies.

Set boundaries: Learn to say no to unnecessary commitments and prioritize activities that nourish your mind, body, and soul. Establish boundaries with work, family, and social obligations to protect your time for self-care.

Delegate tasks: Don't be afraid to ask for help and delegate tasks to your partner, family members, or trusted friends. Share parenting responsibilities and household chores to free up time for yourself.

Multi-task mindfully: Look for opportunities to combine self-care activities with other tasks or responsibilities. For example, listen to an audiobook while cooking dinner, or practice mindfulness while taking a walk with your children.

Practice self-compassion: Be kind to yourself and let go of perfectionism. Accept that it's okay to prioritize your own needs and take breaks when you need them. Give yourself permission to rest and recharge without guilt.

Seeking Support and Building Resilience

Parenting can be challenging, and it's essential to seek support and build resilience to navigate the ups and downs effectively. Here are some ways to seek support and build resilience as a parent:

Reach out to your support network: Lean on friends, family members, and other parents for support and encouragement. Share your experiences, seek advice, and offer mutual support to one another.

Join parent groups: Connect with other parents through parent groups, online forums, or local support groups. Surround yourself with a supportive community of parents who understand the joys and challenges of raising children.

Attend parenting classes or workshops: Take advantage of parenting classes or workshops that offer guidance and support on topics such as child development, discipline, and self-care. Learn new strategies and techniques for managing parenting stress and building resilience.

Practice self-reflection: Take time to reflect on your parenting journey and identify areas where you can grow and improve. Practice self-awareness and self-compassion, and be willing to learn from your mistakes and adapt your approach as needed.

Seek professional help if needed: If you're struggling with overwhelming stress, anxiety, or depression, don't hesitate to seek professional help from a therapist or counselor. A mental health professional can provide guidance, support, and coping strategies to help you navigate parenting challenges more effectively.

Prioritize self-care rituals: Incorporate self-care rituals into your daily routine to nurture your physical, mental, and emotional well-being. Whether it's a morning meditation practice, an evening bubble bath, or a weekly date night with your partner, prioritize activities that recharge and rejuvenate you.

By seeking support from your network, practicing self-reflection, and prioritizing self-care rituals, you can build resilience and navigate the challenges of parenting with grace and confidence.

Conclusion

As you reach the end of this parenting guide, take a moment to reflect on your journey as a parent. Parenthood is a remarkable journey filled with ups and downs, challenges and triumphs, laughter and tears. It's a journey of growth, learning, and unconditional love, where every day brings new opportunities for connection, growth, and discovery. As you reflect on your parenting journey, consider the following points:

Reflecting on Your Parenting Journey

Think back to the day you became a parent—the excitement, the joy, the sense of wonder and responsibility. Consider how much you've grown and evolved since that moment, as you've navigated the joys and challenges of raising a child. Reflect on the moments that have brought you the most joy—the first smile, the first steps, the laughter and silliness that fill your home. Cherish those memories and hold them close to your heart.

But parenthood is not without its challenges. It's also a journey marked by sleepless nights, tantrums, and moments of doubt and uncertainty. Reflect on the times when you've struggled—the moments when you've felt overwhelmed, exhausted, or unsure of yourself. Acknowledge the challenges you've faced and the lessons you've learned along the way.

Continuing to Meet Your Child's Evolving Needs

As your child grows and develops, so too do their needs and interests. Parenthood is a journey of continuous growth and adaptation, as you strive to meet your child's evolving needs and support their development every step of the way. Reflect on how your parenting approach has evolved over time, as you've learned more about your child's unique personality, strengths, and challenges.

Moving forward, commit to continuing to meet your child's evolving needs with love, patience, and compassion. Stay attuned to your child's cues and signals, and be open to adjusting your parenting approach as needed to support their growth and well-being. Remember that parenting is not a one-size-fits-all endeavor—what works for one child may not work for another. Embrace the uniqueness of your child and celebrate their individuality.

As you continue on your parenting journey, remember to prioritize self-care and seek support when needed. Take time to nurture your own well-being, so you can show up as the best parent you can be for your child. And remember that you're not alone—lean on your support network, seek guidance from trusted sources, and know that there are resources available to help you navigate the challenges of parenthood.

In closing, embrace the joys, challenges, and opportunities that parenthood brings. Cherish the moments of connection, growth, and love that fill your days, and know that your love and dedication are shaping the future of your child in ways both seen and unseen. As you continue on your parenting journey, may you find joy, fulfillment, and endless blessings in the beautiful adventure of raising a child.

Congratulations on your

journey as a parent, and may

the road ahead be filled with

love, laughter, and endless

possibilities.

www.ingramcontent.com/pod-product-compliance
Lightning Source LLC
Chambersburg PA
CBHW070956250726
48663CB00002B/250